Purposeful Power

A 60-Day Journey to Healing,
Discipline, and Spiritual Growth

Chiquita Gale

Dedication

To my four beautiful children—
You are my greatest motivation, my constant reminder of God's grace, and the reason I choose strength every day.
May you always know that you are deeply loved, fiercely protected, and endlessly capable of walking in your own God-given purpose.

To every man and woman who has ever felt broken, unseen, or unworthy—
This is for you.
May these words remind you that your story is not over, and your power is being restored one step, one prayer, one act of faith at a time.

Acknowledgments

First and foremost, I give all glory to God—the One who carried me through seasons I thought would break me, and the One who turned my pain into purpose. Without Him, none of this would be possible.

To my children—thank you for loving me through my imperfect days, for inspiring me to rise when I felt like falling, and for showing me what unconditional love truly looks like.

To my family and friends who prayed for me, checked on me, and reminded me of who I am when I struggled to remember—your love and encouragement have been a lifeline.

To every reader holding this book—thank you for trusting me with a place in your journey. Your willingness to lean into faith and discipline inspires me to keep going. I pray these pages bless you, strengthen you, and remind you that you are never walking alone.

And to those whose names aren't written here but whose impact lives in my heart—you know who you are. I am forever grateful.

Table of Contents

Part One: Foundations of Faith and Fitness

Prologue: Purposeful Power

I didn't ask for this journey—truthfully, I never imagined my life would take this path. But purpose has a way of finding us in the middle of our pain.

There was a time when I felt completely undone. A time when the silence in my home was deafening, and the weight of being a widow and raising four children alone pressed heavily on my chest. Sleepless nights blurred into exhausting days, and I often questioned how I'd make it through the next hour—let alone the next season of my life. But even in the thickest darkness, God has a way of sending light.

I remember mornings where simply getting out of bed felt like a miracle. The grief was heavy. The loneliness louder than I could bear. The enemy whispered that I was finished, that I was too broken to rebuild. But God—gracious and steady—kept drawing me close.

Healing didn't come all at once. There was no thunderous breakthrough moment—just small, surrendered steps. I started handing my pain to God piece by piece. In stillness. In prayer. In those quiet, unfiltered moments with my Bible open and my heart cracked wide.

And somewhere along the way, I realized: I couldn't just wait for healing to arrive. I had to participate in it. I had to move. I had to trust Him enough to take one intentional step, and then another. So, I planned—not just to survive, but to become stronger. In faith. In body. In purpose.

Fitness became my offering. Every drop of sweat was a prayer. Every workout was an act of worship. With every repetition, I was declaring, "I'm still here." I began to feel the parallel between physical resistance and spiritual growth—how both require pressure, but both produce strength.

Abstinence. Boundaries. Fasting. Discipline. These weren't just lifestyle choices—they were spiritual tools. And the more I committed, the more I could feel God rebuilding me from the inside out.

That's when I found it—**Purposeful Power**. Not the kind that impresses others, but the kind that sustains you when no one is watching. The kind that says, "God, I trust You even here." A power rooted not in perfection, but in the presence of a loving Father who knows how to restore.

I wrote this for anyone who's ever asked, "Can I come back from this?" For the woman (or man) who feels stuck. For the person who keeps showing up, even with trembling hands. For the soul who's ready to heal but unsure how to begin.

This book isn't a fitness manual. Aside from the Bible, it's a lifeline. A companion. A blueprint for healing, discipline, and holy confidence.

You don't need to be perfect to begin. You just need to say yes —
yes to growth, yes to faith, yes to the version of you that God is calling forth.

You are not broken beyond repair. You are being rebuilt for something greater.

The Rebuild: Changes & Sacrifices for True Healing

True healing requires intentional changes and sacrifices. To truly rebuild, I had to confront what was holding me back and commit to letting go of what no longer served God's purpose for me.

Changes I Had to Make:

- Prioritizing My Faith
- Developing a Fitness Routine
- Creating Healthy Boundaries
- Practicing Abstinence
- Consistent Prayer & Reflection
- Shifting My Mindset
- Choosing Forgiveness
- Avoiding Secular Music & Harmful Content
- Filling My Mind with God's Truth

Sacrifices I Had to Make for Healing:

- Letting Go of Comfort
- Giving Up Immediate Gratification
- Denying the Flesh
- Breaking Free from Emotional Attachments
- Prioritizing Time with God
- Rebuilding Self-Worth
- Choosing Purposeful Content

Purposeful Reflections:

1. What changes do I need to make to align my life with God's purpose for me?
2. What sacrifices am I avoiding that are necessary for my healing?
3. What thoughts, music, or content do I need to remove from my life to help me become who God called me to be?
4. Who do I need to forgive, and what areas of my heart need healing?
5. What steps can I take today to rebuild my life with Purposeful Power?

_____

_____

_____

_____

_____

_____

_____

_____

_____

_____

_____

_____

_____

_____

_____

Healing in Motion: How Movement Restores the Mind

"Breathe in grace. Exhale control."
Healing isn't just something you think your way into—it's something you move through. Every stretch, every step, every bead of sweat is a conversation between your body and your spirit. Movement gives your pain a pathway to leave and makes room for peace to enter.

When you move, you remind yourself that you're still alive, still capable, and still chosen. Don't chase perfection in your workouts—pursue presence. Let each breath become prayer.

Breathing Exercise:
Inhale: "God, fill me with Your peace."
Exhale: "I release what I can't control."

Affirmation:
"I move not to fix myself, but to free myself."

Introduction: Walking in Purposeful Power

This book is not just about workouts or checklists—it's about spiritual renewal, mental resilience, and physical discipline rooted in faith. You've already taken a significant step by opening this book, and I want to walk alongside you for the next 60 days as you commit to becoming more intentional with your growth.

Purposeful Power is structured in four key parts:

- **Foundations of Faith and Fitness** – where we establish the mindset, habits, and spiritual alignment needed to begin well.
- **Strength in Purpose and Discipline** – where you'll reflect on the changes and sacrifices required to grow stronger inside and out.
- **Strength for the Body. Faith for the Soul.** – featuring your daily workouts and faith challenges to guide your transformation.
- **Reflection and Commitment** – where you'll look back, reflect, and prepare to carry *Purposeful Power* beyond the page.

Throughout this journey, you'll be encouraged to reflect regularly using the **Purposeful Reflections** pages. These are opportunities for you to connect what's happening in your body with what's stirring in your soul.

You'll also notice the intentional inclusion of scriptures, prayers, and reflection space to help you stay grounded in your walk with God while honoring your temple.

This isn't about perfection—it's about faithfulness. There will be challenges, but there will also be breakthroughs. There will be resistance, but there will also be results. If you're willing to show up—God will meet you right where you are.

Now, let's begin with open hearts, surrendered minds, and expectant spirits. You're not just entering a program—you're stepping into purpose.

Formation of Habit: The Key to Lasting Discipline

"No discipline seems pleasant at the time, but painful. Later, however, it produces a harvest of righteousness and peace for those who have been trained by it." – **Hebrews 12:11**

Success in both **faith and fitness** is not about feelings or motivation—it is about **habits**. *Purposeful Power* is designed to help you shift from inconsistency to **intentional discipline**, training your mind, body, and spirit to operate in alignment with God's purpose for you.

Why Habits Matter

A habit is a **routine behavior** that, when repeated consistently, becomes second nature. Many people struggle to stay committed to their goals because they rely on **motivation**, which comes and goes. But **discipline, powered by consistent habits, creates lasting transformation**.

Just as you don't wake up physically strong overnight, you don't develop spiritual or mental strength in a day. It takes **intentional, daily effort** to form habits that align with your purpose.

The Three Keys to Habit Formation

1. Start with Intention

Every habit begins with a **decision**. You must commit to showing up daily, whether it's in prayer, movement, or mindset shifts.

✓ **Morning and Nighttime Prayers** set the foundation for your discipline.

✓ **Scheduling your workouts** removes excuses and builds consistency.

✓ **Daily reflections** help reinforce purpose and keep you accountable.

2. Make it Simple & Repeatable

If a habit feels overwhelming, it's less likely to stick.

✓ Set **specific, small goals** instead of vague ones (e.g., "Pray every morning before touching my phone" vs. "Pray more").

✓ Anchor new habits to existing routines (e.g., stretching while listening to scripture).

✓ Remove obstacles—**set out your workout clothes, place your Bible by your bedside, and plan ahead**.

3. Be Consistent, Not Perfect

Transformation happens through **repetition, not perfection**.

✓ **When you miss a day, don't quit—start again.**

✓ **Track your progress**—even small wins add up.

✓ **Pray for discipline** when you don't feel motivated.

Faith, Fitness, and the Power of Habits

✓ When you make **prayer a habit**, your faith deepens.

✓ When you make **exercise a habit**, your body strengthens.

✓ When you make **discipline a habit**, your purpose unfolds.

By the end of these **60 days**, your habits will shape a **stronger, more focused, and more spiritually disciplined version of yourself**. This is not just a program—it's a **lifestyle shift**.

Are you ready to build **habits that align with your purpose**?

Introductory Prayer: Aligning Your Journey with God

"Commit your works to the Lord, and your plans will be established." –
Proverbs 16:3

Before we begin, it's important to recognize the **power of prayer** in transforming our journey. Prayer is the **foundation** that connects us to God, aligns our intentions with His purpose, and strengthens our resolve.

By beginning this journey with **prayer**, we invite God to:
✓ **Guide us with wisdom** and clarity.
✓ **Provide strength** to remain disciplined.
✓ **Align our actions** with His will.
✓ **Remind us that we are not alone**, for His presence is our greatest source of support and encouragement.

Let this first prayer serve as a **spiritual jumpstart**, setting the tone for the **60 days ahead**.

Prayer for Strength, Discipline, and Purpose

Heavenly Father,

I come before You today, surrendering this journey into Your hands. I acknowledge that without You, my strength is limited, but with You, all things are possible. Lord, I ask for discipline—discipline to remain consistent, to push past doubt, and to stay committed to both my faith and my fitness. Let my body be a vessel for Your work, and may my actions bring glory to You.

As I embark on these 60 days, help me to stay focused. When I feel weak, be my strength. When distractions arise, remind me of my purpose. When I am tempted to quit, fill me with the endurance to persevere. Lord, align my heart, my mind, and my body with Your will. Let this journey be more than just a transformation—I want it to be a testimony of Your power in my life.

Thank You for this opportunity to grow in faith, fitness, and discipline. I trust that through this process, you will shape me into the person You have called me to be. I move forward in faith, with purpose, and in Your strength.

Amen.

A Journey Rooted in Faith

This is more than a fitness plan—it's a commitment to **spiritual and physical renewal**. As you **pray daily**, stay **disciplined in your actions**, and **trust God's process**, you will not only see change—you will **become stronger in faith and purpose**.

Daily Prayers: Establishing Discipline Through Prayer

Making Prayer a Forethought, Not an Afterthought

Prayer is a powerful tool, not just for spiritual connection, but for **discipline, focus, and consistency**. Prayer is your soul's resistance training — It builds spiritual endurance with every repetition.

The goal of these daily prayers is to help you:

✓ **Make prayer a natural part of your routine** – not a last-minute thought.
✓ **Train your mind and spirit for discipline** – just as you train your body.
✓ **Strengthen your focus** – keeping faith and fitness aligned as priorities.
✓ **Develop resilience** – overcoming distractions and staying committed.

These prayers are structured to be your **foundation**—helping you start and end each day with the right mindset.

Morning Prayer: Strength, Focus, and Discipline

Scripture Reference: *"Commit your works to the Lord, and your plans will be established."* – **Proverbs 16:3**

Prayer:

Heavenly Father,

I thank You for this new day and the strength You have given me. Today, I commit my body, mind, and spirit to You. Strengthen my discipline so that I remain consistent in my faith and fitness journey. Keep my thoughts aligned with Your will, and help me overcome distractions, fatigue, or doubt. Give me endurance for the challenges ahead and wisdom to make choices that honor

You. I declare that today I walk in focus, power, and purpose. Thank You for guiding me every step of the way.

Amen.

Nighttime Prayer: Reflection, Gratitude, and Renewal

Scripture Reference: *"In peace I will lie down and sleep, for You alone, Lord, make me dwell in safety."* – **Psalm 4:8**

Prayer:

Heavenly Father,

As this day comes to an end, I pause to thank You for every lesson, every challenge, and every victory. I repent for any distractions or moments of weakness that pulled me away from my purpose. Forgive me for anything I may have done that was not in alignment with Your will. I surrender my thoughts, worries, and plans to You tonight, trusting that You will give me rest and renewal for tomorrow. Continue to shape my discipline and strengthen my faith as I grow closer to You.

Amen.

Why Daily Prayer Matters for Discipline

Prayer Strengthens Habit Formation

- Just like training in fitness, the more consistently you pray, the more natural it becomes. **Discipline is about consistency, not convenience.**

Prayer Keeps You Focused on Your Goals

- Life is full of distractions, but daily prayer helps you **reset your mind** and **stay aligned** with your faith and fitness journey.

Prayer Prepares Your Spirit for Strength

- Just as a warm-up prepares your body, prayer prepares your **mind, body, and spirit** for the challenges ahead.

Prayer Cultivates Gratitude and Awareness

- A lifestyle of prayer shifts your mindset from frustration to **gratitude and purpose**, reminding you why you started.

By making **daily prayer a disciplined habit**, you train your **mind, body, and spirit** to walk in alignment with faith and fitness—ensuring that your journey is not just about results, but about building a **strong foundation of consistency, strength, and obedience**.

Healing in the Midst of Turmoil

"He heals the brokenhearted and binds up their wounds." – **Psalm 147:3**

There are seasons when healing doesn't feel holy—it feels heavy. When the prayers seem unanswered, the tears don't stop, and you wonder if God still sees you. But even in those moments, He is working beneath the surface, rearranging what once felt shattered into something sacred.

Healing isn't always loud. Sometimes it's the quiet decision to try again, pray again, move again, and believe again. It's learning to find God not only in the victory, but also in the vulnerability.

This section is for the days that stretch your faith—the moments when you don't feel strong, but you still show up. Because that's where true transformation happens **in the midst of turmoil.**

When God Feels Silent

"Be still, and know that I am God." – **Psalm 46:10**

There will be moments when heaven feels quiet. You'll pray and hear nothing. You'll ask and see no movement. But silence is not absence—it's often the sacred space where God shapes endurance. He is still speaking, even when you can't hear the words. His silence is a sign that something deeper is taking root.

Divine Insight:
What might God be strengthening in me when I can't hear Him speaking?

Learning to Forgive Yourself

"Though your sins are like scarlet, they shall be as white as snow." – **Isaiah 1:18**

Forgiving others is hard. Forgiving yourself can feel impossible. Yet, holding on to shame only delays the healing God wants to give. You are not the mistakes you made—you are the testimony He's creating. Grace is not earned; it's received. Let go of guilt and agree with God's mercy over your life.

Divine Insight:
What would change in my heart if I truly believed I am already forgiven?

Letting Go of Control

"Trust in the Lord with all your heart and lean not on your own understanding." – **Proverbs 3:5**

Control often disguises fear. We hold on tightly because we're afraid of what will happen if we don't. But faith asks us to release, to trust that even when the plan shifts, God's promise doesn't. When you loosen your grip, you make room for grace.

Divine Insight:
What fear am I still holding onto that keeps me from resting in God's peace?

Part Two: Strength in Purpose and Discipline

Purposeful Power: Finding Purpose in Being Fit & Faithful

True strength comes not just from lifting weights or enduring long workouts, but from aligning our purpose with God's will. When we understand that our bodies are sacred vessels for His work, we find deeper motivation to stay committed to faith and fitness.

Why Purpose Matters

When we act with purpose, discipline becomes less about restriction and more about fulfillment. Living fit and faithful is not about vanity or mere self-improvement—it is about stewardship. When we care for our bodies, we honor God's creation. When we build strength, we equip ourselves to serve others more effectively.

Think of an athlete training for a marathon. Without a clear goal, their training feels pointless. But with a finish line in sight, every step has meaning. Likewise, when we anchor our fitness and faith journey in purpose, we develop the endurance needed to stay committed even when challenges arise.

How to Cultivate Purpose in Faith and Fitness

- **Shift Your Mindset** – Instead of seeing fitness as a chore, view it as an opportunity to glorify God with your body.
- **Set Intentional Goals** – Aim for goals that align with both faith and health (e.g., completing 60 days of scripture-based workouts).
- **Rely on God's Strength** – On difficult days, remind yourself that God equips you for every challenge. You are not alone in this journey.
- **Use Your Strength for Good** – Being strong isn't just about aesthetics; it's about having the endurance to serve, lead, and live a life pleasing to God.

Scriptures for Discipline and Purposeful Mindset

- *Do you not know that your bodies are temples of the Holy Spirit, who is in you, whom you have received from God? You are not your own; you*

- *were bought at a price. Therefore, honor God with your bodies.* (**1 Corinthians 6:19-20**)
- *Whatever you do, work at it with all your heart, as working for the Lord, not for human masters.* (**Colossians 3:23**)
- *For physical training is of some value, but godliness has value for all things, holding promise for both the present life and the life to come.* (**1 Timothy 4:8**)
- *Be transformed by the renewing of your mind. Then you will be able to test and approve what God's will is—His good, pleasing, and perfect will.* (**Romans 12:2**)
- *I discipline my body and keep it under control, lest after preaching to others I myself should be disqualified.* (**1 Corinthians 9:27**)

By grounding ourselves in God's word and seeing fitness as an act of faith, we transform the way we approach discipline. Every workout, every healthy choice, and every prayer brings us closer to His purpose for our lives.

Avoiding Distractions and Overcoming Temptation

Discipline is not just about what we do; it's about why we do it. The strength to stay committed to faith and fitness comes from having a deep understanding of our **why**—the purpose behind our actions. When distractions arise and temptation pulls at us, our **why** is what keeps us anchored.

Why Your "Why" Matters

Without a strong reason, it's easy to falter. When we lack clarity, distractions become excuses, and temptations feel justifiable. A strong why gives us the mental and spiritual endurance to push through challenges.

Consider these examples:

- **Faith:** If your goal is to grow spiritually, knowing that time spent in prayer and scripture strengthens your relationship with God will help you prioritize devotion over social media or unnecessary distractions.
- **Fitness:** If your why is to be healthy for your children, remembering that skipping workouts or indulging in unhealthy habits could impact your longevity will motivate you to stay committed.
- **Lifestyle:** If you're working towards financial freedom, avoiding impulsive spending will be easier when you remind yourself that every wise financial decision builds the legacy you want to leave.

Recognizing Distractions and Temptations

21

Distractions often come disguised as good things that keep us from **greater** things. Temptations appeal to our immediate desires but often compromise our long-term goals.

Common Distractions:

- Excessive screen time (social media, TV, texting) – *"Be very careful, then, how you live—not as unwise but as wise, making the most of every opportunity, because the days are evil."* – **Ephesians 5:15-16**
- Procrastination (convincing yourself you'll start tomorrow) – *"The sluggard does not plow in the autumn; he will seek at harvest and have nothing."* – **Proverbs 20:4**
- People who discourage or pull you away from your purpose – *"Do not be misled: 'Bad company corrupts good character.'"* – **1 Corinthians 15:33**
- Overcommitting to activities that drain rather than enrich you – *"Martha, Martha,"* the Lord answered, *"you are worried and upset about many things, but few things are needed—or indeed only one."* – **Luke 10:41-42**
- Materialism and the love of money – *"For the love of money is a root of all kinds of evil."* – **1 Timothy 6:10**
- Worry and anxiety – *"Therefore do not worry about tomorrow, for tomorrow will worry about itself."* – **Matthew 6:34**
- Seeking human approval over God's approval – *"Am I now trying to win the approval of human beings, or of God? Or am I trying to please people? If I were still trying to please people, I would not be a servant of Christ."* – **Galatians 1:10**
- Idolatry – *"You shall have no other gods before me."* – **Exodus 20:3-4**
- Pride and self-reliance instead of trusting God – *"Pride goes before destruction, a haughty spirit before a fall."* – **Proverbs 16:18**

Common Temptations:

- Skipping workouts when feeling unmotivated – *"A little sleep, a little slumber, a little folding of the hands to rest—and poverty will come on you like a thief and scarcity like an armed man."* – **Proverbs 24:33-34**
- Giving in to unhealthy cravings despite your fitness goals – *"Do not join those who drink too much wine or gorge themselves on meat, for drunkards and gluttons become poor, and drowsiness clothes them in rags."* – **Proverbs 23:20-21**
- Neglecting prayer or scripture because of a busy schedule – *"But seek first his kingdom and his righteousness, and all these things will be given to you as well."* – **Matthew 6:33**

- Dwelling on negativity or engaging in gossip rather than maintaining a positive, faith-filled mindset – *"Do not let any unwholesome talk come out of your mouths, but only what is helpful for building others up according to their needs."* – **Ephesians 4:29**
- Lust and sexual immorality – *"Flee from sexual immorality. All other sins a person commits are outside the body, but whoever sins sexually, sins against their own body."* – **1 Corinthians 6:18**

How to Stay Focused and Resilient

- **Write down your why** – Keep it visible as a daily reminder.
- **Pray for strength** – Ask God for guidance in moments of weakness.
- **Eliminate unnecessary distractions** – Set boundaries with time and commitments.
- **Surround yourself with like-minded individuals** – Accountability is key.
- **Replace temptation with purpose** – When faced with temptation, turn to an alternative action aligned with your goals (e.g., scripture reading instead of social scrolling, a quick workout instead of skipping altogether).

Scriptural Support

- *"Set your minds on things above, not on earthly things."* – **Colossians 3:2**
- *"No temptation has overtaken you except what is common to mankind. And God is faithful; he will not let you be tempted beyond what you can bear."* – **1 Corinthians 10:13**

Your **why** is your foundation. The stronger your why, the harder it is for distractions or temptations to shake you. Stay disciplined, stay focused, and always move with purpose.

Purposeful Reflection:

- What distractions have held you back in past fitness or faith journeys?
- How can you turn those distractions into opportunities for spiritual and physical growth?
- Which scripture will you hold onto when facing temptation?

Unforgiveness: A Weight Even the Strongest Can't Carry

You can train your body to carry heavy things — but some weights can't be lifted with muscle. Unforgiveness is one of them.

No matter how disciplined, focused, or physically strong you become, carrying the weight of unforgiveness will eventually break you down — from the inside out.

It's the invisible burden that tightens your chest, shortens your breath, and weakens your peace. You can stretch, sweat, and strengthen every muscle in your body, but if your heart stays clenched in bitterness, your spirit will never move freely.

Forgiveness isn't a sign of weakness — it's proof of spiritual strength.
It takes courage to release what hurt you, maturity to let go of what you can't change, and faith to believe that God can heal what others broke.

Think of it like a weighted vest: it adds resistance, but it's not meant to be worn forever. You build strength *by* carrying resistance, but you find freedom *when you remove it.*

Unforgiveness slows your spiritual progress. It drains energy you could be using to love, build, and grow. And just like a body under too much pressure, your spirit eventually gives out under the weight of what it was never meant to hold.

When you choose forgiveness, you choose to drop the weight. You make space for God's peace to flow again — for joy, creativity, and clarity to return.

Letting go doesn't mean forgetting. It means freeing your heart to move forward unrestrained. Forgiveness releases you — not them.

Scripture Focus:
*"Bear with each other and forgive one another if any of you has a grievance against someone. Forgive as the Lord forgave you." — **Colossians 3:13 (NIV)***

Purposeful Reflection:
What weight have I been carrying that no longer serves my healing?
What would it look like to hand that weight to God today?

The Importance of the Sabbath Day of Rest

The Sabbath is a divine commandment and a gift from God, meant to provide rest and renewal. Observing the Sabbath is crucial not only spiritually but also emotionally, mentally, and physically.

1. **Spiritually:** It is a day set apart for worship and reflection, drawing us closer to God.
   - *"Remember the Sabbath day, to keep it holy."* – **Exodus 20:8**
   - *"Then he said to them, 'The Sabbath was made for man, not man for the Sabbath.'"* – **Mark 2:27**
2. **Emotionally:** Resting on the Sabbath allows for emotional reset, reducing stress and promoting inner peace.
   - *"Come to me, all who labor and are heavy laden, and I will give you rest."* – **Matthew 11:28**
3. **Mentally:** Stepping away from daily tasks and distractions sharpens our focus and renews our minds.
   - *"Be still and know that I am God."* – **Psalm 46:10**
4. **Physically:** The human body was designed to need rest, and the Sabbath provides the perfect opportunity for recovery and rejuvenation.
   - *"In six days, the Lord made heaven and earth, and on the seventh day he rested and was refreshed."* – **Exodus 31:17**

Honoring the Sabbath is an act of obedience and faith, acknowledging God as our provider. It allows us to reset, realign, and reconnect with what truly matters.

Fasting: Strengthening Your Spirit & Body

"But when you fast, put oil on your head and wash your face,
so that it will not be obvious to others that you are fasting,
but only to your Father, who is unseen;
and your Father, who sees what is done in secret, will reward you."
— **Matthew 6:17–18**

Fasting is more than giving something up — it's *making room for God*.

Before beginning this 60-day journey, fasting allows you to quiet distractions, align your heart, and renew your focus. It's an intentional act of surrender — laying down physical desires to strengthen spiritual discipline.

The Purpose of Fasting Before a Workout Plan

Starting a fitness journey with a fast is a declaration:

"God, I'm not doing this by my strength — I'm doing it through Yours."

Fasting before you begin helps you:

- **Reset your focus.** It reminds your body and mind that the goal isn't appearance — it's alignment with God's will.
- **Detox your habits.** You begin your plan with a cleansed body and a clear mind.
- **Break emotional and physical dependencies.** When you feel hungry or tempted, you learn to rely on prayer instead of impulse.
- **Rebuild spiritual sensitivity.** When your body quiets, your spirit listens more deeply.

Fasting is a way to prepare not only your muscles, but your mindset.

Before You Begin: How to Approach a Fast

If you've never fasted before, start small and focus on intention, not deprivation.
Here are a few types of fasts that fit within a faith + fitness journey:

Daniel Fast	21 days of fruits, vegetables, nuts, grains, and water (no meat, sugar, or processed foods)	7–21 days
Intermittent Fast	Set eating windows (e.g., 8 hours of eating, 16 hours of fasting)	3–7 days to start
Social Media or Distraction Fast	Abstain from entertainment, gossip, or anything that steals focus from God	Entire 60 days or specific weeks
Juice or Liquid Fast	Only fresh juices, smoothies, or soups (ensure nutritional balance)	1–3 days (great pre-reset before Week 1)

💡 *Important:* **Always consult a medical professional before fasting if you have health conditions, are pregnant, or on medication.**

Benefits of Fasting During a Workout Plan

Fasting during your fitness journey can yield powerful **spiritual and physical benefits** when done with balance and prayer:

Spiritual Benefits

- Deepens prayer life and focus.
- Increases gratitude and humility.
- Builds endurance and self-control — a reflection of true discipline.
- Opens spiritual clarity — your spirit becomes more aware of God's guidance.

Physical Benefits

- Aids in detoxification and improves metabolism.
- Helps reduce inflammation and bloating.
- Promotes fat loss while preserving lean muscle (with proper nutrition).
- Increases energy and focus after the adjustment period.

Expectations and Boundaries During Fasting

Expectations:

- The first few days may feel uncomfortable — tiredness, irritability, or cravings are normal.
- Your energy may dip temporarily before stabilizing.
- You may feel emotional — fasting brings hidden things to the surface so healing can begin.

Boundaries:

- Stay hydrated — water and electrolytes are essential.
- Break your fast gently with nourishing, whole foods.
- Don't push your body to exhaustion; pair fasting with rest and stretching when needed.
- Listen to your body and the Holy Spirit — both will tell you when to slow down or adjust.

Pros and Cons of Fasting During a Workout Plan

Strengthens self-discipline and spiritual focus	Can cause fatigue or dizziness if overdone
Promotes metabolic and hormonal balance	May hinder muscle recovery if calorie intake is too low
Reduces cravings and resets appetite	Can lead to burnout if combined with excessive workouts
Improves mental clarity and emotional balance	May affect hormones in women if not managed properly
Teaches reliance on God's strength	Requires wisdom and prayer — not performance

Remember: Fasting is not about perfection — it's about **presence**. The goal is not to prove your strength, but to draw closer to the One who provides it.

Fasting Prayer

Heavenly Father,

I enter this time of fasting to realign my heart with Yours. As I quiet the noise and still my desires, speak clearly to me. Give me strength to discipline my body and renew my spirit. Let this fast prepare me for the physical and spiritual work ahead. May every hunger pang remind me to hunger for You.

In Jesus' name, Amen.

Divine Insight:

What area of my life is God asking me to surrender before I begin this journey?

Pre-Workout Prayer

Purpose of the Prayer: A pre-workout prayer is a moment to center yourself, inviting God into your fitness journey. It sets the tone for discipline, focus, and gratitude, acknowledging that your strength comes from Him. This prayer helps you overcome mental barriers, distractions, and fatigue while aligning your fitness goals with spiritual purpose.

Prayer:

Heavenly Father,

Thank You for the body You have given me, a temple to honor and serve You. As I prepare for this workout, I ask for strength, endurance, and focus. Keep me free from distractions and help me push through any obstacles with perseverance. Let this session be an act of discipline and self-care, glorifying You in all I do.

I rebuke any thoughts of doubt, fatigue, or discouragement, replacing them with courage and determination. May this workout not only strengthen my body but also my mind and spirit. Help me remain humble, patient, and committed to my journey of health and wellness.

Let Your presence be with me, guiding my movements and renewing my energy. I trust in Your power, Lord, to sustain me and push me beyond my limits in a way that honors You. In Jesus' name, I pray. Amen.

Part Three: Strength for the Body. Faith for the Soul.

60-Day Workout Plan Overview

Purpose of the Plan: The 60-day workout plan is designed to build consistency, discipline, and strength, both physically and mentally. By committing to this structured routine, you will enhance endurance, increase muscle tone, and reinforce the habit of movement as an act of self-care and gratitude. Each workout integrates faith-based motivation to keep you focused on your why.

Workout Breakdown

The plan is divided into two phases:

Phase 1: Weeks 1-4 (30-Minute Workouts)

These workouts focus on foundational strength, endurance, and form. The goal is to establish consistency and prepare the body for increased intensity.

Weekly Routine:

- **Day 1:** Full-Body Strength Training (Squats, Push-ups, Crunches, Planks)
- **Day 2:** Cardio Endurance (Sit-Ups, High Knees, Burpees, Sprints)
- **Day 3:** Active Recovery & Mobility (Stretching, Yoga, Core Activation)
- **Day 4:** Upper Body & Core (Push-ups, Shoulder Press, Triceps Dips, Russian Twists)
- **Day 5:** Lower Body & Glutes (Lunges, Deadlifts, Calf Raises, Squat Pulses)
- **Day 6:** Cardio & Agility (Box Jumps, Mountain Climbers, Jump Squats, Ladder Drills)
- **Day 7:** Rest & Reflection (Scripture Reading, Meditation, Gentle Stretching)

WEEK 1 - COMMITTING TO THE JOURNEY

DEVOTIONAL: TAKING THE FIRST STEP

Theme: Obedience & Commitment
Scripture: *"Commit to the Lord whatever you do, and he will establish your plans."* — **Proverbs 16:3 (NIV)**

Faith Check-In:

Every journey begins with a decision. The hardest part of any fitness or faith transformation is committing to it. When you surrender your journey to God, you're inviting Him to guide your steps and give you the strength to stay consistent.

Prayer:

Father, I dedicate this journey to You. Strengthen my heart, body, and mind to stay committed, even when challenges arise. Lead me in faith and fitness as I take this first step. Amen.

WORKOUT PLAN: WEEK 1 - BUILDING CONSISTENCY

Focus: Establishing a solid foundation in discipline, movement, and faith.

Day 1: Foundational Strength

Warm-up: 5 minutes of stretching or light cardio

Circuit (3 Rounds):
• 10 Bodyweight Squats (Modified: Assisted Squats | Advanced: Jump Squats)
• 10 Push-ups (Modified: Knee Push-ups | Advanced: Diamond Push-ups)
• 20-second Plank (Modified: Knees Down | Advanced: One-Leg Plank)
• 15 Lunges (Each Leg)

Faith Challenge: Meditate on Proverbs 16:3 (Commit to the Lord whatever you do, and He will establish your plans.) before starting.

Purposeful Reflection: What fears or doubts do I have about this journey? How can I trust God to guide me through them?

Day 2: Cardio & Core

Warm-up: 5-minute brisk walk or light jog

Circuit (3 Rounds):
• 30-second High Knees
• 10 Sit-ups (Modified: Crunches | Advanced: Weighted Sit-ups)
• 20 Bicycle Crunches
• 1-minute Plank Hold (can be broken into 2 x 30 seconds)

Faith Challenge: Read and reflect on Philippians 4:13 (I can do all things through Christ who strengthens me.)

Purposeful Reflection: What are some obstacles I've overcome in the past? How can those experiences help me now?

_____

_____

_____

_____

_____

_____

_____

_____

_____

_____

Day 3: Active Recovery (Sabbath & Stretching)

Stretching & Prayer: Spend time in active rest. Stretch your muscles, do light yoga, or take a peaceful walk.

Faith Challenge: Meditate on Exodus 20:8 (Remember the Sabbath day and keep it holy.)

Purposeful Reflection: How can I invite God into my moments of rest?

_____

_____

_____

_____

_____

_____

_____

_____

_____

_____

_____

_____

_____

_____

Day 4: Upper Body & Endurance

Warm-up: Arm circles, shoulder rolls, light jogging

Circuit (3 Rounds):
• 10 Triceps Dips (Chair/Bench)
• 12 Shoulder Press (Dumbbells or Water Bottles)
• 10 Bicep Curls
• 30-second Jump Rope (or Jumping Jacks)

Faith Challenge: Thank God for the ability to move. Meditate on 1 Corinthians 6:19-20 (Your body is a temple of the Holy Spirit).

Purposeful Reflection: What does honoring my body as a temple of God mean to me?

_____

_____

_____

_____

_____

_____

_____

_____

_____

_____

Day 5: Lower Body Strength

Warm-up: 5-minute stair climb or walking lunges

Circuit (3 Rounds):
- 12 Squats (Hold Dumbbells if Advanced)
- 10 Glute Bridges
- 15 Calf Raises
- 30-second Wall Sit

Faith Challenge: Before starting, reflect on Hebrews 12:11 (No discipline seems pleasant at the time, but later it produces a harvest of righteousness).

Purposeful Reflection: Where in my life do I need more discipline? How can I invite God into those areas?

_____

_____

_____

_____

_____

_____

_____

_____

_____

_____

Day 6: Full-Body Endurance

Warm-up: 5-minute jog

Circuit (3 Rounds):
- 15 Burpees
- 12 Push-ups
- 20 Mountain Climbers
- 1-minute Jump Rope

Faith Challenge: Pray for strength to endure hard moments in fitness and faith. Meditate on Isaiah 40:29 (He gives strength to the weary and increases the power of the weak.)

Purposeful Reflection: When have I felt spiritually weak? How did God strengthen me?

_____

_____

_____

_____

_____

_____

_____

_____

_____

Day 7: Reflection & Rest

Active Recovery: Go on a nature walk, stretch, and reflect.

Faith Challenge: Reflect on how God sustained you this week. Meditate on Psalm 46:10 (Be still and know that I am God).

Purposeful Reflection: What are three blessings I experienced this week?

_____

_____

_____

_____

_____

_____

_____

_____

_____

_____

_____

_____

_____

_____

WEEK 2 - DEVELOPING DISCIPLINE

DEVOTIONAL: PUSHING THROUGH TEMPTATION

Theme: Strength in Obedience

Scripture: *"No temptation has overtaken you except what is common to mankind. And God is faithful; he will not let you be tempted beyond what you can bear."* — **1 Corinthians 10:13 (NIV)**

Heart Posture:

The enemy will tempt you with excuses, distractions, and fatigue, but God has given you the strength to resist. Discipline is built through daily decisions to stay faithful to the journey.

Prayer:

Lord, help me resist the temptation to quit. Strengthen my discipline and help me push forward with determination. Amen.

WORKOUT PLAN: WEEK 2 – ENDURANCE & FAITH

Focus: Building physical and spiritual stamina through consistency.

Day 1: Foundational Strength – Stability & Control

Warm-up: 5 min dynamic stretching (arm swings, hip openers, bodyweight squats)

Circuit (3 Rounds):
• 12 Squats (Modified: Sit to Stand | Advanced: Jump Squats)
• 10 Push-ups (Modified: Wall Push-ups | Advanced: Elevated Feet)
• 20 Crunches
• 30-Second Plank

Faith Challenge: Meditate on **Galatians 6:9** – *"Let us not become weary in doing good…"*

Purposeful Reflection: Am I staying consistent in the small things, trusting they lead to transformation?

_____

_____

_____

_____

_____

_____

_____

_____

_____

_____

_____

_____

_____

_____

_____

_____

Day 2: Cardio Endurance – Heart & Hustle

Warm-up: 3 mins jogging in place + dynamic lunges

Circuit (3 Rounds):
• 25 High Knees (Each Leg)
• 15 Sit-ups
• 12 Burpees
• 40-Second Sprint (or Power Walk if modifying)

Faith Challenge: Meditate on **Hebrews 12:1** – *"Let us run with perseverance the race marked out for us."*
Purposeful Reflection: What is weighing me down that I need to surrender?

_____

_____

_____

_____

_____

_____

_____

_____

_____

_____

_____

_____

_____

Day 3: Active Recovery & Core Connection

Routine:
- 5 Minutes Light Stretching
- 5-Minute Yoga Flow (Cat-Cow, Downward Dog, Warrior II)
- 3 Rounds of Core Activation:
- 10 Bird Dogs
- 15 Glute Bridges
- 30-Second Side Planks

Faith Challenge: Meditate on **Psalm 23:3** – *"He refreshes my soul..."*
Purposeful Reflection: How can I make rest a holy, intentional practice?

_____

_____

_____

_____

_____

_____

_____

_____

_____

_____

_____

_____

Day 4: Upper Body & Core Focus

Warm-up: Arm Circles + Jumping Jacks (3 minutes)

Circuit (3 Rounds):
• 12 Push-ups
• 10 Dumbbell Shoulder Press (or water bottles)
• 15 Triceps Dips
• 25 Russian Twists

Faith Challenge: Meditate on **Ephesians 6:10** – *"Be strong in the Lord and in His mighty power."*
Purposeful Reflection: Where do I need more spiritual strength? How can I pray for it?

_____

_____

_____

_____

_____

_____

_____

_____

_____

_____

_____

Day 5: Glutes & Lower Body

Warm-up: March in place + standing hamstring stretch

Circuit (3 Rounds):
• 15 Reverse Lunges
• 10 Dumbbell or Bodyweight Deadlifts
• 25 Calf Raises
• 15 Squat Pulses

Faith Challenge: Meditate on **Psalm 119:133** – *"Direct my footsteps according to your word."*
Purposeful Reflection: How can I walk more purposefully in obedience this week?

_____

_____

_____

_____

_____

_____

_____

_____

_____

_____

_____

_____

Day 6: Cardio & Agility Boost

Warm-up: Jump rope or light jog (3 minutes)

Circuit (3 Rounds):
• 10 Box Jumps or Step-Ups
• 20 Mountain Climbers
• 15 Jump Squats
• 20 Seconds of Ladder Drills or Quick Feet

Faith Challenge: Meditate on **Philippians 4:13** – *"I can do all things through Christ..."*
Purposeful Reflection: What challenge this week can I face head-on with God's strength?

_____

_____

_____

_____

_____

_____

_____

_____

_____

_____

_____

Day 7: Rest & Reflect

Activity:
• Gentle Full Body Stretch (10 minutes)
• Read or listen to scripture
• Meditate & journal

Faith Challenge: Meditate on **Psalm 46:10** – *"Be still and know that I am God."*
Purposeful Reflection: What progress have I made? Where have I seen God move?

_____

_____

_____

_____

_____

_____

_____

_____

_____

_____

_____

_____

_____

WEEK 3 - STRENGTH & ENDURANCE

DEVOTIONAL: STRENGTH IN DISCIPLINE

Theme: Overcoming Laziness
Scripture: *"The soul of the sluggard craves and gets nothing, while the soul of the diligent is richly supplied."* — **Proverbs 13:4 (ESV)**

Journey Review:

Discipline is not just about motivation; it's about commitment. There will be days when you don't feel like working out or praying. But success doesn't come from feelings—it comes from consistency. God rewards diligence, whether in faith or fitness. When you show up, even on tough days, you build strength both spiritually and physically.

Prayer:

Heavenly Father, give me the strength to remain disciplined even when I feel weak. Help me to push through distractions and tiredness. May my efforts honor You, and may I see the fruits of consistency in my faith and fitness journey. Amen.

WORKOUT PLAN: WEEK 3 - STRENGTH & ENDURANCE

Day 1: Foundational Strength – Core Stability

Warm-up: 5 minutes of marching in place + shoulder rolls

Circuit (3 Rounds):
• 15 Squats (Modified: Sit to Stand | Advanced: Weighted Squats)
• 12 Push-ups
• 20 Crunches
• 30-Second Forearm Plank

Faith Challenge: Meditate on **1 Corinthians 3:11** – *"For no one can lay any foundation other than the one already laid, which is Jesus Christ."*

Purposeful Reflection: How am I building my life on Christ in this season?

Day 2: Cardio Endurance – Next Level Push

Warm-up: Jog in place or jump rope (3 minutes)

Circuit (3 Rounds):
• 20 High Knees
• 10 Burpees
• 15 Sit-Ups
• 45-Second Sprint or Fast Feet

Faith Challenge: Meditate on **Psalm 18:29** – *"With your help I can advance against a troop..."*

Purposeful Reflection: What limits have I accepted that God is calling me to break?

_____

_____

_____

_____

_____

_____

_____

_____

_____

_____

Day 3: Active Recovery & Stretch Reset

Routine:
- 10-Minute Flow:
- – Child's Pose → Cat/Cow
- – Low Lunge (each side)
- – Supine Twist
- – Deep Breathing

Core Activation (Optional 2 rounds):
- 10 Bird Dogs
- 15 Glute Bridges
- 20 Second Plank

Faith Challenge: Meditate on **Isaiah 30:15** – *"In repentance and rest is your salvation..."*

Purposeful Reflection: What area of my life needs rest or reset?

_____

_____

_____

_____

_____

_____

_____

_____

_____

Day 4: Upper Body & Core

Warm-up: Arm swings + Jumping Jacks (3 minutes)

Circuit (3 Rounds):
- 10 Push-ups
- 10 Dumbbell Shoulder Press
- 12 Triceps Dips
- 30 Russian Twists

Faith Challenge: Meditate on **Proverbs 31:17** – *"She sets about her work vigorously; her arms are strong for her tasks."*

Purposeful Reflection: What daily "task" do I need strength and grace for?

_____

_____

_____

_____

_____

_____

_____

_____

_____

_____

Day 5: Lower Body & Glutes Burn

Warm-up: Leg swings, lunges, light jogging (5 minutes)

Circuit (3 Rounds):
- 12 Lunges (Each Leg)
- 10 Deadlifts
- 30 Calf Raises
- 20 Squat Pulses

Faith Challenge: Meditate on **Psalm 37:23** – *"The Lord makes firm the steps of the one who delights in him."*

Purposeful Reflection: What does it look like to let God order my steps?

_____

_____

_____

_____

_____

_____

_____

_____

_____

_____

Day 6: Cardio & Agility Challenge

Warm-up: Light jump rope (2 min) + Dynamic Stretches

Circuit (3 Rounds):
• 12 Box Jumps or Step-Ups
• 20 Mountain Climbers
• 15 Jump Squats
• 30-Second Agility Ladder or Side-to-Side Shuffle

Faith Challenge: Meditate on **Habakkuk 3:19** – *"The Sovereign Lord is my strength..."*
Purposeful Reflection: How does agility in fitness relate to flexibility in life and faith?

_____

_____

_____

_____

_____

_____

_____

_____

_____

_____

_____

Day 7: Rest & Recharge

Activity:
• 10 Minutes of Gentle Movement or Prayer Walk
• Read, reflect, or write a gratitude list

Faith Challenge: Meditate on **Psalm 62:1** – *"Truly my soul finds rest in God..."*

Purposeful Reflection: What am I thankful for in my journey so far?

_____

_____

_____

_____

_____

_____

_____

_____

_____

_____

_____

_____

_____

_____

WEEK 4 - ENDURANCE & FAITHFULNESS

DEVOTIONAL: PERSEVERING IN FAITH & FITNESS

Theme: Faithfulness in Small Things
Scripture: *"Whoever can be trusted with very little can also be trusted with much."* — **Luke 16:10 (NIV)**

Pause and Praise:

Small steps lead to big changes. God sees our faithfulness in the little things—our commitment to prayer, to movement, to honoring our bodies. Whether you run one mile or walk for ten minutes, consistency is key.

Prayer:

Lord, help me to remain faithful in the small moments, knowing that they prepare me for greater things. Strengthen my endurance in both my spiritual and fitness journeys. Amen.

WORKOUT PLAN: WEEK 4 - ENDURANCE CHALLENGE

Day 1: Foundational Strength – Full Body Flow

Warm-up: 5 minutes of dynamic body movement

Circuit (3 Rounds):
• 15 Squats
• 10 Push-ups
• 20 Crunches
• 30-Second Plank
• 12 Lunges

Faith Challenge: Meditate on **Romans 12:2** – *"Be transformed by the renewing of your mind…"*
Purposeful Reflection: What new mindset am I stepping into?

_____

_____

Day 2: Cardio Endurance – Spiritual Drive

Warm-up: Jog or shadowbox (3 minutes)

Circuit (3 Rounds):
• 25 High Knees
• 15 Sit-ups
• 12 Burpees
• 45-Second Sprint or Lateral Shuffle

Faith Challenge: Meditate on **Jeremiah 29:11** – *"For I know the plans I have for you..."*

Purposeful Reflection: Am I moving like someone with purpose and destiny?

_____

_____

_____

_____

_____

_____

_____

_____

_____

_____

_____

_____

Day 3: Active Recovery & Flexibility

Routine:
• 10-Minute Flow: Deep hip stretches, spinal twists, hamstring + quad stretches
• 2 Rounds of:
– Bird Dogs
– Supine Breathing
– Core Engagement Holds

Faith Challenge: Meditate on **John 14:27** – *"Peace I leave with you..."*
Purposeful Reflection: How am I making room for peace, not pressure?

_____

_____

_____

_____

_____

_____

_____

_____

_____

_____

_____

_____

_____

Day 4: Upper Body & Core Burnout

Warm-up: Jump rope + Arm Swings (3 minutes)

Circuit (3 Rounds):
• 12 Push-ups
• 12 Shoulder Press
• 15 Triceps Dips
• 30 Russian Twists
• 20 Second Plank

Faith Challenge: Meditate on **Philippians 1:6** – *"He who began a good work in you..."*

Purposeful Reflection: Where do I see progress that I once prayed for?

_____

_____

_____

_____

_____

_____

_____

_____

_____

_____

_____

Day 5: Lower Body & Glutes Finish Strong

Warm-up: March in place + Leg Swings + Bodyweight Squats

Circuit (3 Rounds):
• 15 Lunges
• 12 Deadlifts
• 30 Calf Raises
• 15 Squat Pulses
• 10 Glute Bridges

Faith Challenge: Meditate on **Job 17:9** – *"The righteous keep moving forward..."*
Purposeful Reflection: How can I keep moving forward even on tough days?

_____

_____

_____

_____

_____

_____

_____

_____

_____

_____

_____

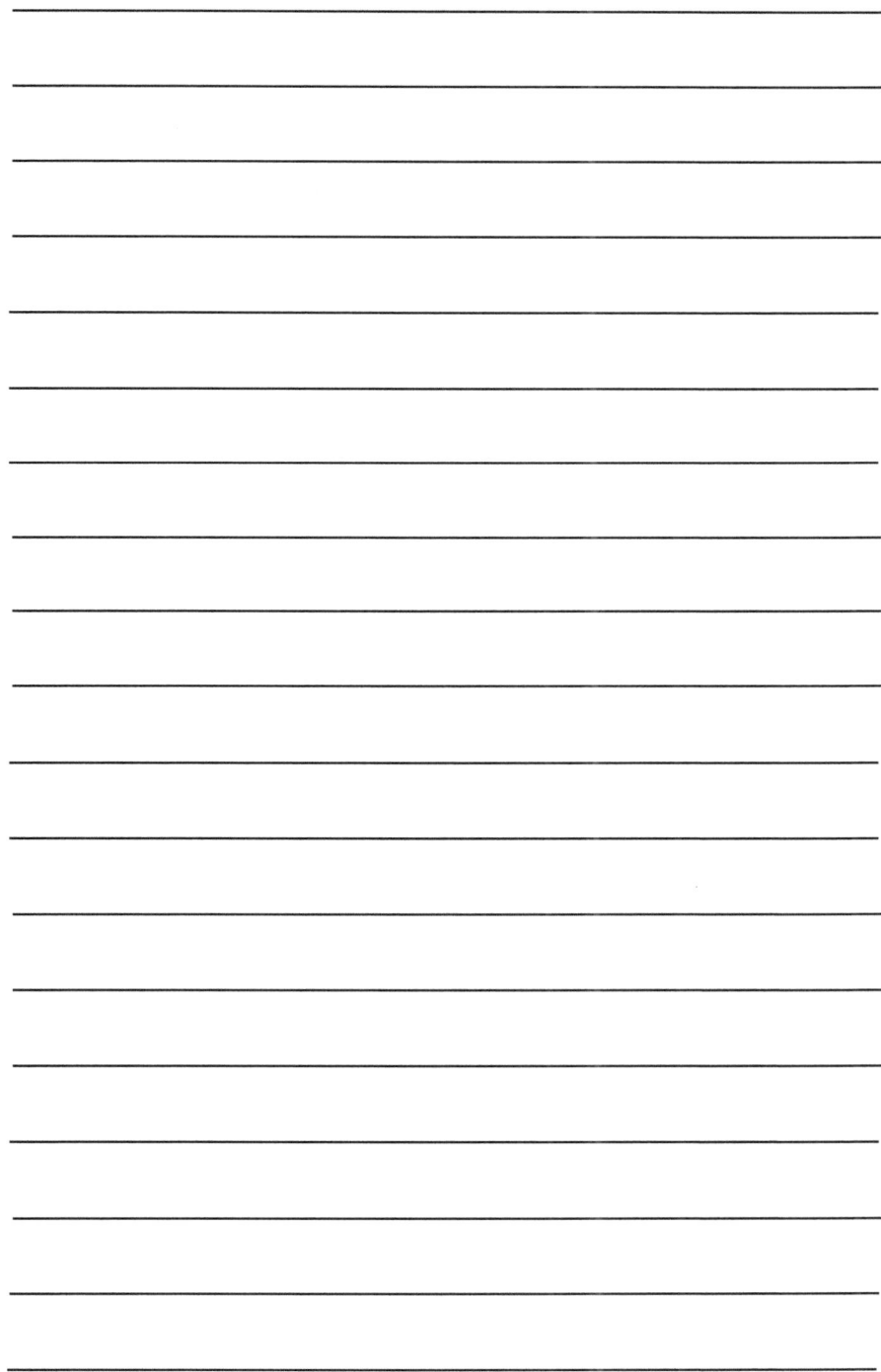

Day 6: Cardio & Agility – Push to the Finish

Warm-up: Jog or Jumping Jacks (3 minutes)

Circuit (3 Rounds):
• 15 Box Jumps
• 25 Mountain Climbers
• 20 Jump Squats
• 30 Seconds of Quick Feet or Ladder Drills

Faith Challenge: Meditate on **Joshua 1:9** – *"Be strong and courageous…"*

Purposeful Reflection: What does courage look like for me right now?

_____

_____

_____

_____

_____

_____

_____

_____

_____

_____

Day 7: Rest & Reflection

Activity:
• Prayer Walk, Journaling, or Gratitude Flow
• Full Body Stretch (10 minutes)

Faith Challenge: Meditate on **Psalm 91:1** – *"Whoever dwells in the shelter of the Most High..."*

Purposeful Reflection: How has God covered me in this journey?

_____

_____

_____

_____

_____

_____

_____

_____

_____

_____

_____

_____

_____

Phase 2: Weeks 5-8 (1-Hour Workouts)

Workouts intensify to build endurance and challenge the body further. Strength and conditioning take priority.

Weekly Routine:

- **Day 1:** Strength Training & Core (Deadlifts, Chest Press, Hanging Leg Raises, Planks)
- **Day 2:** High-Intensity Interval Training (HIIT) (Kettlebell Swings, Sprint Intervals, Burpees)
- **Day 3:** Mobility & Recovery (Foam Rolling, Yoga, Deep Stretching)
- **Day 4:** Upper Body Strength (Pull-ups, Bench Press, Dumbbell Shoulder Press, Core Work)
- **Day 5:** Lower Body Power (Bulgarian Split Squats, Hip Thrusts, Box Jumps)
- **Day 6:** Endurance & Speed (Long-Distance Running, Circuit Training, Agility Drills)
- **Day 7:** Sabbath Rest & Reflection (Prayer Walk, Journaling, Gratitude Practices)

WEEK 5 – LEVEL UP: MIND, BODY & SPIRIT

DEVOTIONAL: STRENGTH FOR THE JOURNEY

Theme: Rising to the Challenge
Scripture: *"Have I not commanded you? Be strong and courageous. Do not be afraid; do not be discouraged..."* — **Joshua 1:9 (NIV)**

Victory Thoughts:
You've laid the foundation—now it's time to build. This week, challenge yourself. New strength requires new effort. As your workouts intensify, so should your spiritual endurance. God is with you in every rep.

Prayer:
Father, Thank You for the strength You've already given me. As I stretch beyond my limits this week, help me trust you for even more. Empower my body, renew my mind, and keep my spirit focused on You. Amen.

Day 1: Full-Body Power Circuit

Warm-up (10 min): Jump rope, dynamic stretches, arm/leg swings

Circuit (4 Rounds):
- 15 Squats (Weighted if possible)
- 15 Push-ups
- 20 Sit-Ups or V-Ups
- 1-Minute Plank
- 20 Alternating Lunges
- 10 Burpees

Cool-down: Deep breathing + full-body stretch (5 min)
Faith Challenge: Meditate on Isaiah 41:10

Purposeful Reflection: What does courage look like in my fitness journey this week?

_____

_____

_____

_____

_____

_____

_____

_____

_____

_____

Day 2: HIIT + Core Burn

Warm-up (10 min): Light jog, high knees, shoulder rolls

Workout (4 Rounds):
• 30 Seconds: Jump Squats
• 30 Seconds: Rest
• 30 Seconds: Mountain Climbers
• 30 Seconds: Rest
• 30 Seconds: Russian Twists
• 30 Seconds: Plank to Push-Up
• 1-Minute Sprint or Fast Feet

Finisher (2 Rounds):
• 15 Sit-Ups
• 10 Bicycle Crunches
• 1-Minute Wall Sit

Cool-down: Stretch and hydrate
Faith Challenge: Meditate on Galatians 6:9

Purposeful Reflection: Where am I tempted to quit, and how can I push through?

_____

_____

_____

_____

_____

_____

_____

_____

Day 3: Active Recovery + Spiritual Alignment

Focus: Mobility, breathing, and core awareness

Flow:
- 10-Minute Breath-Focused Stretching
- 5-Minute Prayer Walk or Journaling
- 3 Rounds of:
– 10 Bird Dogs
– 10 Glute Bridges
– 30-Second Plank
– 5 Deep Belly Breaths

Faith Challenge: Meditate on Psalm 46:1

Purposeful Reflection: How can I use rest as a tool for growth?

_____

_____

_____

_____

_____

_____

_____

_____

_____

_____

Day 4: Upper Body Strength & Core

Warm-up (10 min): Arm circles, light resistance band work, jumping jacks

Circuit (4 Rounds):
- 12 Push-ups
- 12 Dumbbell Shoulder Press
- 12 Bent-Over Rows
- 10 Triceps Dips
- 25 Russian Twists
- 20 Sit-Ups

Cool-down: Stretch arms, back, neck
Faith Challenge: Meditate on Ephesians 6:10

Purposeful Reflection: Where in my life do I need more spiritual strength?

_____

_____

_____

_____

_____

_____

_____

_____

_____

_____

Day 5: Glutes & Lower Body Focus

Warm-up (10 min): High knees, lunges, glute bridges

Circuit (4 Rounds):
• 15 Dumbbell Deadlifts
• 20 Reverse Lunges
• 20 Calf Raises
• 15 Goblet Squats
• 10 Glute Bridges (Hold 5 sec at top)
• 30-Second Wall Sit

Cool-down: Seated hamstring + quad stretches
Faith Challenge: Meditate on Psalm 119:133

Purposeful Reflection: Am I moving with purpose or just going through the motions?

_____

_____

_____

_____

_____

_____

_____

_____

_____

_____

Day 6: Agility + Conditioning Challenge

Warm-up (10 min): Light jump rope, jumping jacks, toe taps

Circuit (4 Rounds):
• 20 Box Jumps (or Step-Ups)
• 15 Jumping Lunges
• 30 Mountain Climbers
• 15 Burpees
• 1-Minute Ladder Drills or Quick Feet
• 1-Minute Sprint

Cool-down: Full-body foam roll or yoga flow
Faith Challenge: Meditate on Philippians 3:14

Purposeful Reflection: What is the "prize" I'm pressing toward—physically and spiritually?

_____

_____

_____

_____

_____

_____

_____

_____

_____

_____

_____

Day 7: Rest & Realignment

Focus: Restoration for body and soul

Activity:
• 20-Minute Stretch or Slow Yoga
• Listen to worship music or a devotional
• Gratitude journaling

Faith Challenge: Meditate on Exodus 33:14

Purposeful Reflection: What do I need to lay down to experience true rest?

_____

_____

_____

_____

_____

_____

_____

_____

_____

_____

_____

_____

WEEK 6 – REFINEMENT THROUGH RESISTANCE

DEVOTIONAL: STRETCHED FOR GREATER

Theme: Growth Comes Through Pressure
Scripture: *"Consider it pure joy… whenever you face trials… because you know that the testing of your faith produces perseverance."* — **James 1:2-3 (NIV)**

Stretch Reflection:
Growth doesn't come without resistance. Just like muscles need to be stretched and stressed to grow stronger, so do our spirits. This week, embrace the pressure. God is shaping you through the stretch.

Prayer:
Lord, when I feel challenged, remind me it's part of the process. Strengthen my heart, my body, and my spirit to rise through resistance. Help me push with purpose and faith. Amen.

Day 1: Full-Body Strength Circuit

Warm-up (10 min): Jog in place, inchworms, dynamic lunges

Circuit (4 Rounds):
• 20 Bodyweight or Dumbbell Squats
• 12 Push-ups
• 15 Dumbbell Rows (Each Side)
• 20 Walking Lunges
• 1-Minute Wall Sit
• 30-Second Plank

Cool-down: Stretch + Deep Breathing
Faith Challenge: Meditate on Isaiah 40:31

Purposeful Reflection: What area of my life needs endurance right now?

Day 2: HIIT Blast + Cardio Core

Warm-up (10 min): Jump rope, high knees, arm circles

HIIT Circuit (5 Rounds, 30/30s):
• Jump Squats
• Mountain Climbers
• Russian Twists
• Burpees
• Fast Feet
• Plank Jacks

Finisher (2 Rounds):
• 15 Sit-Ups
• 20 Bicycle Crunches
• 1-Minute Plank

Cool-down: Full body stretch
Faith Challenge: Meditate on 2 Corinthians 12:9

Purposeful Reflection: How can I let God's strength carry me when mine runs low?

_____

_____

_____

_____

_____

_____

_____

_____

Day 3: Recovery & Realignment

Routine:
• 5-Minute Breathwork
• 10-Minute Flow (Child's Pose, Cat/Cow, Pigeon Stretch, Down Dog, Cobra)
• Core Reset (2 Rounds):
− 10 Dead Bugs
− 10 Glute Bridges
− 1-Minute Seated Stillness

Faith Challenge: Meditate on Matthew 11:28

Purposeful Reflection: What thoughts or tensions do I need to release today?

_____

_____

_____

_____

_____

_____

_____

_____

_____

_____

_____

Day 4: Upper Body Superset

Warm-up (10 min): Shoulder mobility, push-ups, jumping jacks

Circuit (4 Rounds):
- 12 Push-ups
- 12 Shoulder Press
- 10 Bicep Curls (Each Arm)
- 12 Bent-Over Rows
- 10 Triceps Kickbacks
- 25 Russian Twists

Cool-down: Neck, shoulder, and arm stretches
Faith Challenge: Meditate on Philippians 4:13

Purposeful Reflection: Am I giving my full effort, or holding back in any area?

_____

_____

_____

_____

_____

_____

_____

_____

_____

_____

Day 5: Glute & Leg Sculpt

Warm-up (10 min): March in place, glute bridges, leg swings

Circuit (4 Rounds):
- 15 Goblet Squats
- 12 Reverse Lunges
- 10 Romanian Deadlifts
- 20 Calf Raises
- 30 Glute Kickbacks
- 1-Minute Wall Sit

Cool-down: Lower body stretching
Faith Challenge: Meditate on Psalm 18:33

Purposeful Reflection: How am I preparing my steps for greater purpose?

_____

_____

_____

_____

_____

_____

_____

_____

_____

_____

Day 6: Agility + Endurance Challenge

Warm-up (10 min): Jump rope, toe taps, shuffle drills

Agility Circuit (4 Rounds):
• 20 Jumping Lunges
• 30 Mountain Climbers
• 15 Box Jumps or Step-Ups
• 10 Burpees
• 45 Seconds Quick Feet
• 1-Minute Sprint or Speed Walk

Cool-down: Full body stretch & foam roll
Faith Challenge: Meditate on 1 Corinthians 9:24

Purposeful Reflection: What's my "why" for this journey, and how is God using it?

_____

_____

_____

_____

_____

_____

_____

_____

_____

_____

Day 7: Sabbath Stretch & Reset

Activity:
- 20-Minute Stretch + Worship Music
- Gratitude Journal – List 5 Wins This Week
- Read a Devotional or Rest in Nature

Faith Challenge: Meditate on Psalm 91:1

Purposeful Reflection: How did I grow this week—physically, emotionally, spiritually?

_____

_____

_____

_____

_____

_____

_____

_____

_____

_____

_____

_____

_____

WEEK 7 – WALKING IN POWER & PURPOSE

DEVOTIONAL: DISCIPLINE BUILDS DESTINY

Theme: Strengthened by Self-Control
Scripture: *"For the Spirit God gave us does not make us timid, but gives us power, love and self-discipline."* — **2 Timothy 1:7 (NIV)**

Testimony Time:
Discipline is a spiritual tool, not just a physical one. Every time you choose to show up, push through, and honor your temple, you grow in character. This week, tap into God's power and your God-given self-control.

Prayer:
Father, help me to walk boldly in power, love, and self-discipline. Let every rep and every moment of obedience train me for greater things. May I not be ruled by my emotions, but by Your Spirit. Amen.

Day 1: Power Full-Body Strength Circuit

Warm-up (10 min): Jog, arm circles, bodyweight squats

Circuit (4 Rounds):
• 20 Squats (Weighted if possible)
• 12 Push-ups
• 12 Dumbbell Rows
• 20 Walking Lunges
• 30 Second Plank + 10 Push Presses
• 10 Burpees

Cool-down: Deep breathing + full body stretch
Faith Challenge: Meditate on Romans 12:1

Purposeful Reflection: What does it mean to offer my body as a living sacrifice?

_____

_____

Day 2: Explosive HIIT & Core Burnout

Warm-up (10 min): Jump rope, high knees, jumping jacks

HIIT Circuit (5 Rounds):
- 30 Seconds Jump Squats
- 30 Seconds Burpees
- 30 Seconds Mountain Climbers
- 30 Seconds Russian Twists
- 30 Seconds Sprint or Power Walk
- 30 Seconds Rest

Finisher (3 Rounds):
- 15 Sit-ups
- 15 Bicycle Crunches
- 1-Minute Wall Sit

Cool-down: Stretch + Prayer Walk
Faith Challenge: Meditate on Proverbs 25:28

Purposeful Reflection: Where do I need to set better boundaries in my life?

_____

_____

_____

_____

_____

_____

_____

_____

Day 3: Restorative Recovery & Mobility Reset

Routine:
• 5-Minute-Deep Breathing + Prayer
• 10-Minute Stretching Flow (Hips, hamstrings, back, chest)
• 3 Rounds:
– 10 Dead Bugs
– 10 Glute Bridges
– 1-Minute Child's Pose

Faith Challenge: Meditate on Psalm 23:3

Purposeful Reflection: How do I allow God to restore my soul when I feel drained?

_____

_____

_____

_____

_____

_____

_____

_____

_____

_____

_____

Day 4: Upper Body Strength & Stability

Warm-up (10 min): Shoulder rolls, jumping jacks, light band pulls

Circuit (4 Rounds):
• 12 Push-ups
• 12 Dumbbell Shoulder Press
• 10 Dumbbell Rows
• 10 Triceps Dips
• 10 Bicep Curls
• 25 Russian Twists

Cool-down: Arm & chest stretch
Faith Challenge: Meditate on Colossians 3:23

Purposeful Reflection: Am I giving my best effort—spiritually and physically?

_____

_____

_____

_____

_____

_____

_____

_____

_____

_____

Day 5: Glutes, Quads & Hamstrings Builder

Warm-up (10 min): Glute bridges, lunges, jumping jacks

Circuit (4 Rounds):
- 15 Goblet Squats
- 12 Deadlifts
- 20 Step-Ups or Reverse Lunges
- 25 Calf Raises
- 15 Glute Kickbacks
- 30-Second Wall Sit

Cool-down: Hamstring, quad, and glute stretch
Faith Challenge: Meditate on Proverbs 4:26

Purposeful Reflection: How am I preparing for what I'm praying for?

_____

_____

_____

_____

_____

_____

_____

_____

_____

_____

Day 6: Speed, Agility & Endurance Push

Warm-up (10 min): Jog in place, toe taps, shuffle steps

Agility Circuit (4 Rounds):
• 20 Jump Lunges
• 20 Mountain Climbers
• 15 Box Jumps or Step-Ups
• 15 Burpees
• 1-Minute Quick Feet
• 1-Minute Sprint

Cool-down: Stretch or 5-Minute Guided Breathwork
Faith Challenge: Meditate on Hebrews 12:11

Purposeful Reflection: What fruit is being produced in me from staying disciplined?

_____

_____

_____

_____

_____

_____

_____

_____

_____

Day 7: Stillness & Soul Care

Activity:
- 15–20 Minute Walk or Light Stretch with Worship Music
- Read a Psalm or devotional

Faith Challenge: Meditate on Isaiah 26:3

Purposeful Reflection: How can I guard my peace and protect my progress? Where have I seen growth in my faith and fitness since Week 1?

_____

_____

_____

_____

_____

_____

_____

_____

_____

_____

_____

_____

_____

WEEK 8 – FINISHING STRONG WITH FAITH

DEVOTIONAL: THE FRUIT OF YOUR FAITHFULNESS

Theme: Completion with Praise
Scripture: *"I have fought the good fight, I have finished the race, I have kept the faith."* — **2 Timothy 4:7 (NIV)**

Celebration of Growth:
You've shown up, pushed through, and leaned on God. This week, celebrate how far you've come—physically, mentally, and spiritually. It's not about perfection, it's about progress. Faithfulness always produces fruit.

Prayer:
God, thank You for the strength to endure. As I complete this phase, remind me that the discipline I've developed is a testimony to Your faithfulness. I dedicate this final week to You. Finish what You've started in me. Amen.

Day 1: Full-Body Final Challenge

Warm-up (10 min): Jog, dynamic stretches, inchworms

Circuit (5 Rounds):
• 15 Squats (Weighted)
• 15 Push-ups
• 20 Sit-Ups
• 20 Reverse Lunges
• 10 Burpees
• 30-Second Plank

Cool-down: Deep breathing & stretch
Faith Challenge: Meditate on Philippians 1:6
Purposeful Reflection: How has God grown me through this challenge?

_____

_____

_____

_____

Day 2: HIIT & Core Endurance

Warm-up (10 min): Jump rope, high knees, jumping jacks

HIIT Circuit (5 Rounds):
• 30 Seconds Jump Lunges
• 30 Seconds Mountain Climbers
• 30 Seconds Russian Twists
• 30 Seconds Burpees
• 30 Seconds High Knees
• 30 Seconds Rest

Core Finisher (2 Rounds):
• 15 Bicycle Crunches
• 10 Leg Raises
• 1-Minute Plank

Cool-down: Stretch + water
Faith Challenge: Meditate on Galatians 6:9
Purposeful Reflection: Where in my life do I need to continue sowing faithfully?

_____

_____

_____

_____

_____

_____

_____

_____

Day 3: Restorative Recovery & Prayerful Reflection

Routine:
- 10-Minute Full-Body Stretch
- Breathwork & Gratitude Flow
- 2 Rounds of:
– Bird Dogs
– Dead Bugs
– Seated Stillness

Faith Challenge: Meditate on Psalm 103:2
Purposeful Reflection: What am I most grateful for in this journey?

_____

_____

_____

_____

_____

_____

_____

_____

_____

_____

_____

_____

Day 4: Upper Body Strength Test

Warm-up (10 min): Arm swings, shoulder circles, jumping jacks

Circuit (4 Rounds):
- 12 Push-ups
- 12 Dumbbell Shoulder Press
- 12 Bent-Over Rows
- 10 Triceps Dips
- 10 Bicep Curls
- 25 Russian Twists

Cool-down: Upper body stretches
Faith Challenge: Meditate on Proverbs 31:17
Purposeful Reflection: Where do I need to show up strong for myself and others?

_____

_____

_____

_____

_____

_____

_____

_____

_____

_____

_____

Day 5: Glutes & Lower Body Sculpt

Warm-up (10 min): Glute bridges, leg swings, toe touches

Circuit (4 Rounds):
- 15 Goblet Squats
- 20 Reverse Lunges
- 15 Romanian Deadlifts
- 30 Calf Raises
- 15 Glute Kickbacks
- 1-Minute Wall Sit

Cool-down: Foam roll or deep hip & quad stretches
Faith Challenge: Meditate on Psalm 40:2
Purposeful Reflection: How has God kept me grounded through the process?

_____

_____

_____

_____

_____

_____

_____

_____

_____

_____

_____

Day 6: Final Agility & Speed Burnout

Warm-up (10 min): Jog, shuffle drills, jumping jacks

Circuit (5 Rounds):
• 20 Jumping Lunges
• 15 Box Jumps or Step-Ups
• 30 Mountain Climbers
• 1-Minute Sprint
• 10 Burpees
• 45 Seconds Ladder Drills or Quick Feet

Cool-down: Prayer Walk + Stretch
Faith Challenge: Meditate on Isaiah 40:29
Purposeful Reflection: What strength did I discover that I didn't know I had?

_____

_____

_____

_____

_____

_____

_____

_____

_____

_____

_____

Day 7: CELEBRATE, REST & PRAISE

Activity:
• Light walk or joyful movement
• Worship, prayer, or journaling
• Reflect on your testimony of transformation

Faith Challenge: Meditate on Psalm 126:3 – *"The Lord has done great things for us, and we are filled with joy."*
Purposeful Reflection: What's next for me—mentally, spiritually, physically?

_____

_____

_____

_____

_____

_____

_____

_____

_____

_____

_____

_____

_____

_____

Beyond the 60 Days: Maintaining Purposeful Power (7-Day Transition Plan)

1	Gratitude	Write down 10 things God did for you during the 60-day journey.
2	Renewed Vision	Ask: "What does the next level of discipline look like for me?"
3	Rest & Reset	Practice a full Sabbath with no screens—only stillness.
4	Movement with Meaning	Choose one workout that makes you feel powerful.
5	Reconnection	Pray over your goals and ask God to realign your desires.
6	Service	Do one act of kindness or encouragement for someone else.
7	Celebration	Reflect, praise, and plan your "next 30-day chapter."

Part Four: Reflection and Commitment

Spiritual Toolkit: When Distractions Come

Your journey doesn't end here — and neither will the distractions.

This chart is a resource for you to return to when life tries to pull you off track. Use it to pause, pray, and meditate on God's Word as you realign with your purpose.

Let these Scriptures ground you and let the affirmations remind you who you are in Christ.

Distractions, Scriptures, Meditation Thoughts & Affirmations

Distraction	Scripture	Meditation Thought	Affirmation
Tiredness / Low Energy	*Isaiah 40:29* – "He gives strength to the weary and increases the power of the weak."	God supplies strength when yours runs low.	I am filled with God's strength and renewed energy.
Overwhelm / Too Much to Do	*Matthew 11:28-30* – "Come to Me, all who are weary... I will give you rest."	Let God carry the weight — rest is holy.	I find rest and peace in God's presence.
Lack of Motivation	*Galatians 6:9* – "Let us not become weary in doing good…"	Keep sowing seeds — your harvest is coming.	I keep going because my consistency matters.
Negative Self-Talk / Shame	*Romans 8:1* – "There is now no condemnation for those who are in Christ Jesus."	God sees you as loved and forgiven.	I am loved, chosen, and free from condemnation.
Lustful Distractions	*2 Timothy 2:22* – "Flee the evil desires of youth and pursue righteousness…"	Run toward purity and purpose.	I pursue righteousness and honor my body.
Comparison to Others	*Galatians 1:10* – "Am I now trying to win the approval of human beings...?"	Your journey is your own.	I am on my own God-given path.
Discouragement / Setbacks	*Psalm 73:26* – "My flesh and my heart may fail, but God is the strength of my heart…"	Strength is found in God's presence.	I rise again through God's strength.
Family / Friend Drama	*Romans 12:18* – "If it is possible... live at peace with everyone."	Choose peace. Set boundaries.	I protect my peace and walk in love.
Financial Stress	*Philippians 4:19* – "My God will meet all your needs according to His riches…"	God provides — even in lack.	God supplies all my needs in every season.
Temptation to Quit	*Hebrews 12:1-2* – "Let us run with perseverance the race marked out for us…"	Don't quit — fix your eyes on Jesus.	I was built for this. I finish strong.
Poor Time Management	*Ephesians 5:15-16* – "Be very careful, then, how you live... making the most of every opportunity."	Time is a gift — plan with intention.	I manage my time wisely and steward it well.
Feeling Spiritually Disconnected	*James 4:8* – "Draw near to God and He will draw near to you."	God is always one step away.	I reconnect with God today — He is near.

Speak Purposeful Power Over Yourself
(Affirmation Page)

1. I am becoming the woman God created me to be.

2. My discipline is my devotion.

3. My body is a temple; I train it with gratitude.

4. I am not behind; I am being refined.

5. I forgive myself and choose peace.

6. My faith fuels my focus.

7. I am not powerless—I am purposeful.

8. I move with intention, grace, and confidence.

9. God's strength is made perfect in my weakness.

10. I am walking in Purposeful Power.

Closing Thoughts: Walking in Purposeful Power

Take a deep breath.
You made it.

Not just through 60 days of commitment — but through a journey of transformation. You showed up. You pushed through resistance. You prayed when it felt heavy. You moved when it would've been easier to stay still.

And look at you now — standing on the other side of what once seemed impossible.

This is your graduation moment. Not from a school or a program, but from doubt, delay, and distraction. You've completed a journey of discipline and devotion — and that deserves to be celebrated.

You did it — and God did it through you.

This journey wasn't about perfection; it was about perseverance. Every prayer you whispered, every workout you conquered, every reflection you wrote — it all built something eternal inside you. You didn't just strengthen your body; you renewed your spirit. You didn't just finish a challenge; you established a lifestyle of faith, focus, and follow-through.

Now you walk in **Purposeful Power** — not the kind that fades when motivation runs out, but the kind anchored in God's strength.

As you step forward, remember:

- **Healing is holy.** Every scar tells a story of redemption.
- **Discipline is divine.** It's how purpose becomes reality.
- **Movement is ministry.** Each act of endurance glorifies God.

So, celebrate this moment. Praise Him for what He's done *and* for what's still coming.
Because this isn't the finish line — it's the launchpad.

When you feel uncertain, come back to your *Heart Reflections.*
When life feels heavy, return to your *Healing in Motion.*
When you need encouragement, speak your *Affirmations* out loud.
And when you're ready for more, begin *Beyond the 60 Days* — because growth doesn't stop here.

You've crossed the stage. You've earned your strength. You've proven that with God, discipline and devotion can transform your life.

Now go — live boldly, move purposefully, and shine with power.
You are a graduate of perseverance — a living testimony of faith in motion.

"The Lord has done great things for us, and we are filled with joy." — **Psalm 126:3**

About the Author

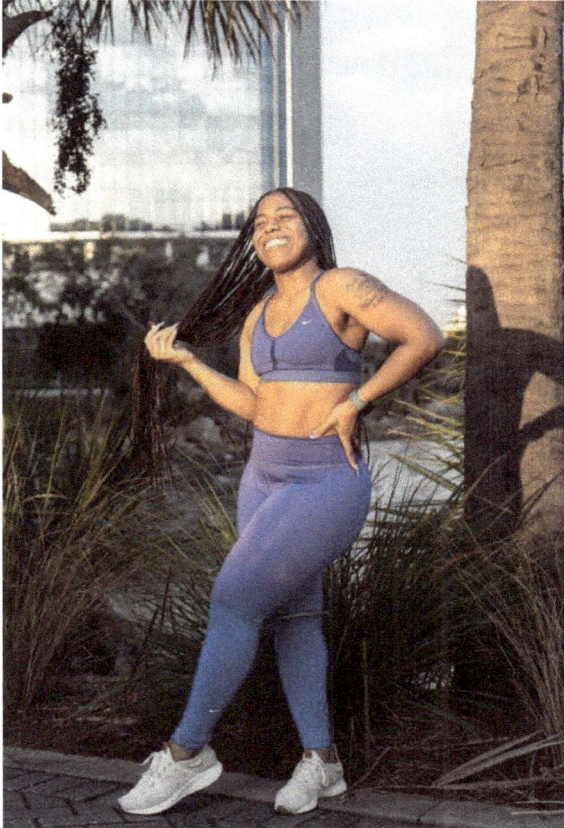

Chiquita Gale is a woman of faith, mother of four, model, and author whose life is a testimony of restoration, resilience, and divine purpose.

With a professional background in **Information Systems** and over a decade of experience in the **IT industry**, Chiquita combines structure, strategy, and spirituality in everything she creates. She holds a **Master's degree in Management Information Systems**, and her analytical mindset, paired with her creative vision, allows her to bridge the gap between technology, transformation, and faith.

After walking through deep loss and seasons of refinement, Chiquita discovered that true strength is built through both movement and mindset. Her journey led her to merge **faith and fitness** — using the body as an instrument of worship and the mind as a space for renewal.

As a model and advocate for holistic healing, she inspires others to live with purpose and confidence — not defined by circumstances but refined by faith. Her heart's mission is to help people see that spiritual discipline and self-care are not separate from success — they are the foundation of it.

Through her **Purposeful Power** brand, Chiquita shares devotionals, resources, and digital content that equip others to heal, grow, and walk boldly in alignment with God's calling.

When she's not writing or creating, you can find her spending time with her children, mentoring others in faith and lifestyle, or developing new ways to inspire personal growth and wellness in the digital space.

Chiquita's life reflects what it means to rebuild from brokenness and rise with grace. Her message is simple yet powerful:

You can renew your mind. You can rebuild your strength. You can walk in Purposeful Power.

Stay connected with Chiquita:
📖 **Website:** www.shopdiamari.com
📷 **Instagram:** @keepitchiq
✉️ **Email:** support@shopdiamari.com

A Note from the Author

Dear Reader,

If you've made it this far, I want to pause and say — *thank you.*

Thank you for showing up for yourself, for trusting this process, and for allowing me to walk alongside you through these pages. Writing *Purposeful Power* was more than a project; it was a prayer. Every word was written with you in mind — to remind you that you are capable of healing, discipline, and divine strength.

This journey wasn't about perfection — it was about progress. You've taken steps that many only talk about taking. You've shown faith in motion, and that's something to be proud of.

I pray that the lessons, scriptures, and reflections in this book continue to guide you long after the final page. May you keep building your habits, protecting your peace, and walking boldly in the purpose God has placed inside you.

If this book blessed you, I'd love to hear your story. Your testimony is powerful — and it could be the encouragement someone else is praying for.

You can connect with me and share your *Purposeful Power Journey* on social media or by email.

Stay steadfast, keep showing up, and remember — every step you take in faith counts.

With love and gratitude,
Chiquita Gale

📖 www.shopdiamari.com
📷 @keepitchiq
✉ support@shopdiamari.com

Scripture quotations are used with permission and are provided solely for the purpose of spiritual study, encouragement, and reflection.

www.ingramcontent.com/pod-product-compliance
Lightning Source LLC
Chambersburg PA
CBHW051246020426
42333CB00025B/3071